DIAGNOSTIC PICTURE TESTS IN

Hypertension

G000077677

DIAGNOSTIC PICTURE TESTS IN

Hypertension

Graham A MacGregor FRCP
Professor of Cardiovascular Medicine,
Blood Pressure Unit
Department of Medicine
St George's Hospital Medical School
London, UK

Ⅳ Mosby-Wolfe

London Baltimore Barcelona Bogotá Boston Buenos Aires Caracas Carlsbad, CA Chicago Madrid Mexico City
Milan Naples, FL New York Philadelphia St. Louis Seoul Singapore Sydney Taipei Tokyo Toronto Wiesbaden

Design & layout:	Lee Riches
Production:	Mary Sketch
Index:	Susan Boobis
Acquisitions Editor:	Claire Hooper

Copyright © 1996 Times Mirror International Publishers Limited.
Published in 1996 by Mosby-Wolfe, a Times Mirror Company.
Originated by Reed Reprographics, Suffolk, UK.
Printed by Grafos S.A. Arte sobre papel, Barcelona, Spain.

ISBN 0 7234 2477 2

For full details of all Times Mirror International Publishers Limited titles, please write to Times
Mirror International Publishers Limited, Lynton House, 7–12 Tavistock Square, London WC1H
9LB, England.

A CIP catalogue record for this book is available from the British Library.

Library of Congress Cataloging-in-Publication Data applied for.

Preface

High blood pressure remains one of the most preventable causes of premature cardiovascular disease. The increasing focus on prevention, investigation and treatment means that most doctors need to have at least some knowledge of this common disorder. I hope these pictures may stimulate an interest to enquire, and to those who are experts, an occasional surprise.

Hypertension is not an easy subject to illustrate. Without the help of my collegues in the Blood Pressure Unit, Dr A.K. Saggar-Malik, Dr C. Missouris, Dr D.R.J. Singer and Mrs N. Markandu, the task would have been very onerous. My grateful thanks to them. I am also indebted to other collegues, in particular to Dr C.M. Corbishley, Dr M.M. Brown, Dr C. Finlayson, Dr A.G. Wilson and Dr M. Feher, for allowing me to use some of their most precious illustrations. Many thanks to them as well.

Graham A. MacGregor
London, 1996

Acknowledgements

The Author and Publisher wish to thank the following individuals, who kindly gave us permission to reproduce their illustrations:

Dr D.H.L. Patterson (Fig. 11, derived from *Diagnostic Picture Tests in Cardiology*); Dr G.R.D. Catto (Figs 13 & 35, derived from *Diagnostic Picture Tests in Renal Disease*); Prof. A.J. Bellingham (Fig. 19, derived from *Diagnostic Picture Tests in Hematology*); Dr M. Parsons (Fig. 32, derived from *Diagnostic Picture Tests in Clinical Neurology*); and Dr S.R. Underwood of the National Heart & Lung Institute, Imperial College of Science, Technology and Medicine, London (Fig. 14).

1 (a) What are the main lesions shown in this digital subtraction renal angiogram? (b) Name three common associated clinical features.

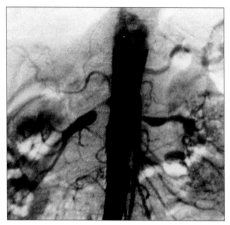

2 The scientist who carried out the first recorded measurement of arterial blood pressure is shown here on the left. (a) Who is he? (b) What did he estimate blood pressure in humans to be?

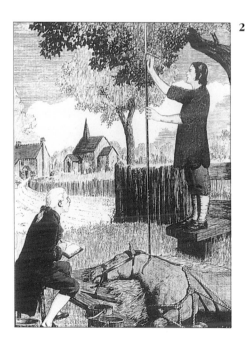

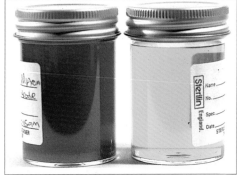

3 One of these two urine specimens, taken from the same patient, has been allowed to stand, the other is fresh.
(a) What is the diagnosis?
(b) What are three common clinical presentations?

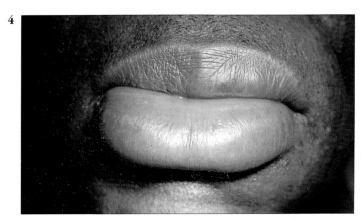

4 This patient with hypertension developed sudden swelling of the lower lip.
(a) What is the diagnosis?
(b) Which class of drug is it almost certainly due to?
(c) Why can it be dangerous ?

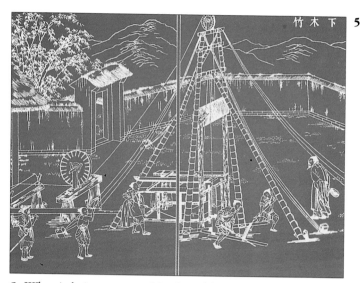

5 What is being extracted in this old print? Who was the first to recognise its relationship to blood pressure?

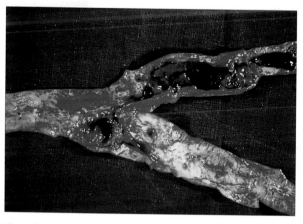

6 (a) What disease process is evident in this carotid artery bifurcation from a patient of 45 years of age?
(b) What are the main preventable predisposing causes?

7

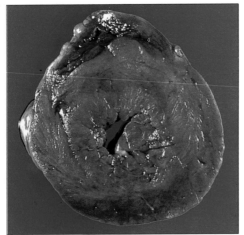

7 (a) What abnormality is seen in this cross-section of a left ventricle?
(b) What is the most likely cause of this abnormality?

8

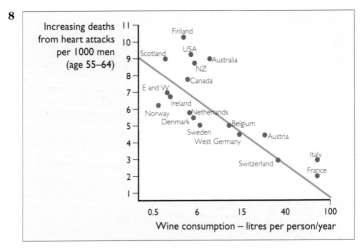

8 What possible mechanisms may explain the relationship between wine consumption and mortality from myocardial infarction, as illustrated in this figure?

9 This is the chest x-ray of a young man with hypertension. What is the arrow pointing to?

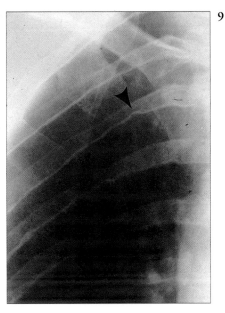

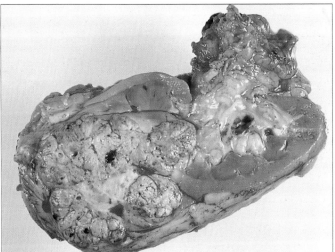

10 What is the lesion shown in this kidney? What is the relationship between this lesion and high blood pressure?

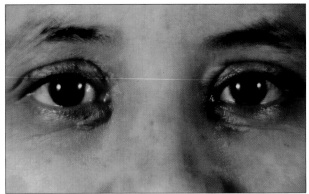

11a

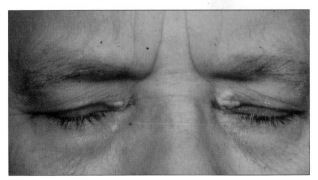

11b

11 The patient in figure **11a** is 25 years old, while the patient in **11b** is 70 years old. Both patients demonstrate the same lesions around the eyes.

(a) What are these lesions called and of what substance are they composed?

(b) Is any other abnormality visible?

(c) What is the significance of these lesions in these patients?

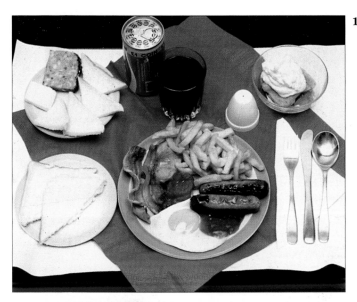

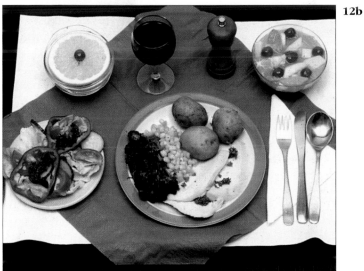

12 What are the relative saturated fat, salt and potassium contents of these two meals?

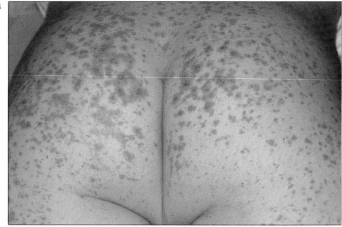

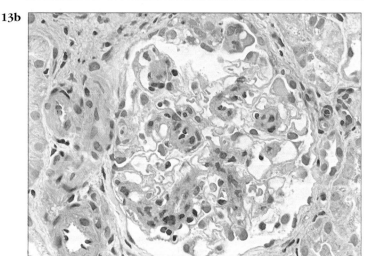

13 These skin lesions (**13a**) occurred in a 10-year-old child.
(a) What is the diagnosis?
(b) What does the renal biopsy (**13b**) show?
(c) What is its association with hypertension?

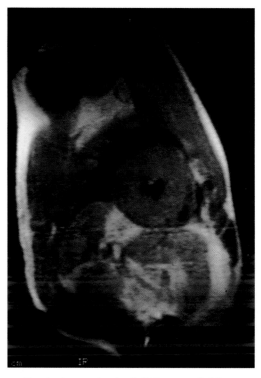

14 What abnormality is shown in the MRI scan of this patient's chest?

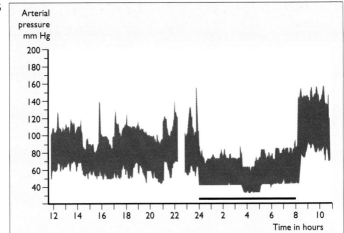

15 What are the possible causes of the high-blood-pressure peaks shown at 16.00 and at 24.00 hours in this ambulatory intra-arterial blood-pressure recording?

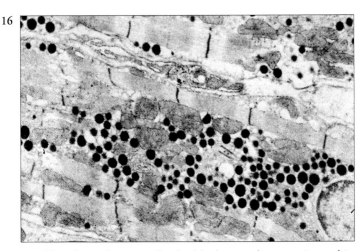

16 (a) What substances do the black granules contain in this electron micrograph of atrial myocytes?
(b) What are the actions of these substances?

17 (a) What does this illustration show?
(b) What class of antihypertensive drugs can cause this side effect and what is the likely mechanism?
(c) What is the best way of treating this side effect?

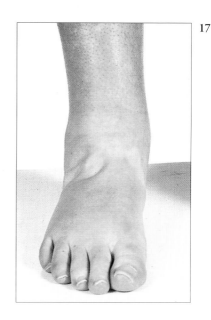

18 This three-dimensional graph shows the results of an important study. What do the results indicate and how are they relevant to the management of hypertension?

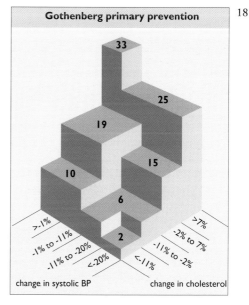

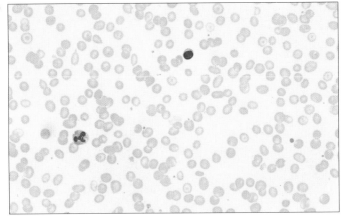

19 This is a blood film from a middle-aged woman with high blood pressure.
(a) What does it show?
(b) What is the probable cause of her high blood pressure?

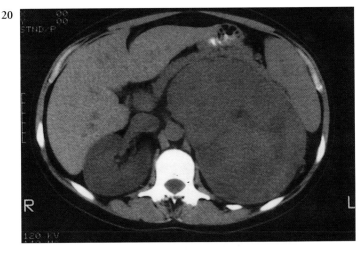

20 What possible diagnosis might be considered in this CT scan of the abdomen of a young woman with hypertension?

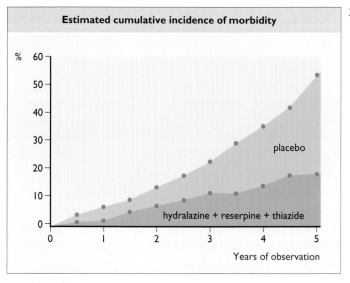

21 This illustrations shows the results of an early study on the effects of treatment of hypertension. Which study is this, which patients did it include and what did the results indicate?

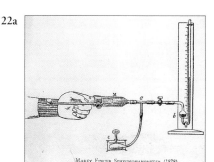

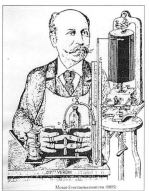

22 These illustrations show two early methods for measuring blood pressure. What was the advantage of using four fingers, rather than one?

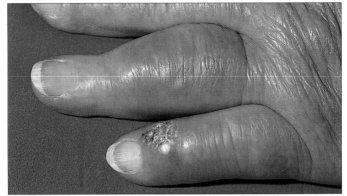

23 This is a photograph of the hand of a 65-year-old woman. What does it show? What class of drugs, used for the treatment of hypertension, may aggravate the symptoms?

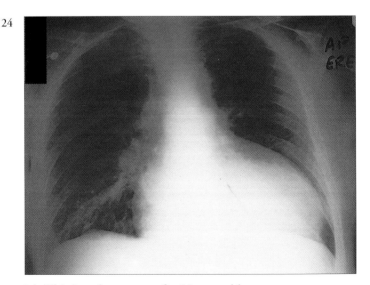

24 This is a chest x-ray of a 55-year-old man.
(a) What does it show?
(b) What are the possible causes?

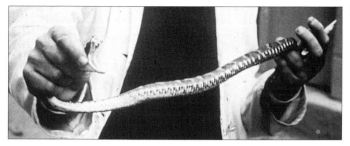

25 What substance was isolated from the Brazilian arrowhead viper (above) which led eventually to a new class of drugs for the treatment of hypertension and heart failure?

26 This tumour, shown whole (**26a**) and in cross-section (**26b**), was removed at laparotomy.
(a) What type of tumour is this?
(b) What is particularly noticeable about this tumour in cross-section?
(c) What symptoms may the patient have exhibited?

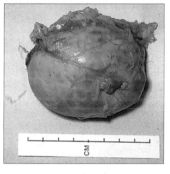

26a

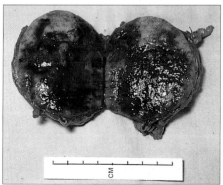

26b

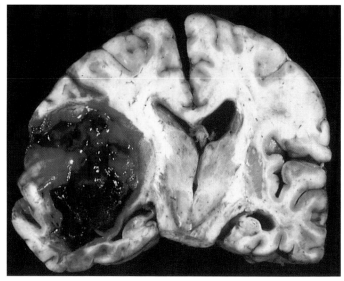

27 What does this cross-section of the brain of a young man show? What is the most likely cause?

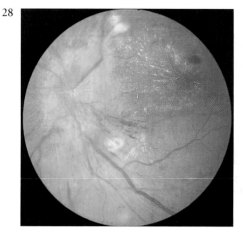

28 What is seen in this retinal photograph? What condition does it indicate?

29 This 55-year-old man had accelerated hypertension, first diagnosed in the 1970s. Which drug has been used to control his blood pressure? Why is this drug now rarely used?

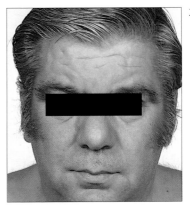

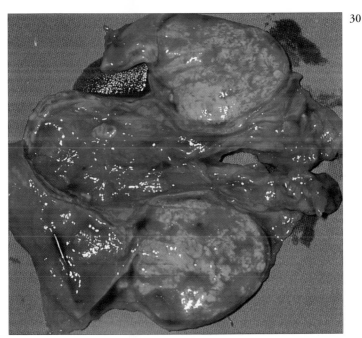

30 What is the lesion shown in this cross-section of an adrenal gland and what condition does it cause? What are the presenting features of this condition? How is the diagnosis confirmed?

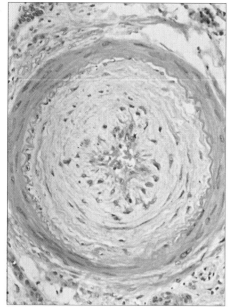

31 This is a cross-section of a renal arteriole.
(a) What is the underlying diagnosis?
(b) What effect does this condition have on renal function?

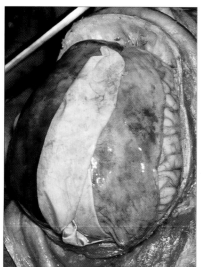

32 (a) What is the lesion shown?
(b) What are the predisposing factors?
(c) What are the common symptoms?

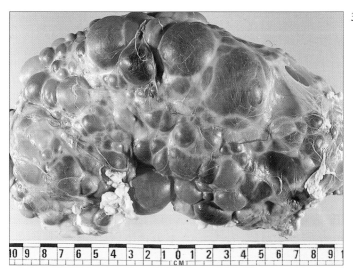

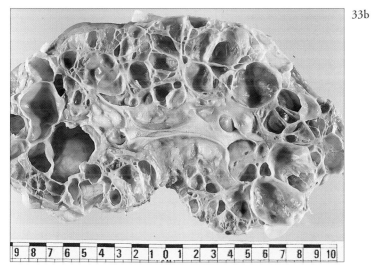

33 (a) What is this condition?
(b) What effect does blood-pressure treatment have on the outcome?

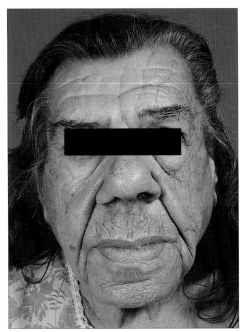

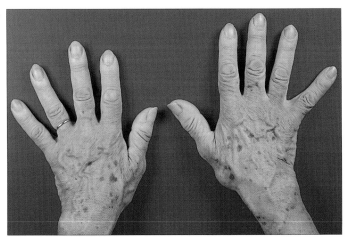

34 (a) What is this condition?
(b) How common is high blood pressure in these patients?

35 (a) What is the congenital abnormality shown?
(b) What complications may develop?

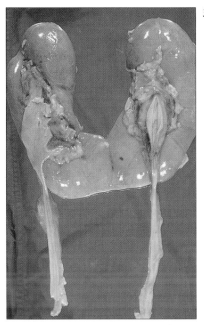

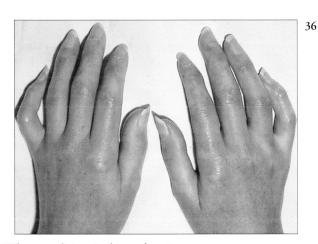

36 (a) What condition is shown here?
(b) What is its relationship to high blood pressure?

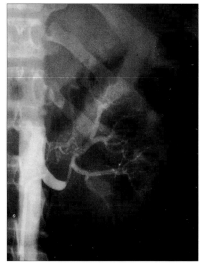

37 These arteriograms are from a young woman with an absent right kidney who suffered from severe hypertension.
(a) What does the arteriogram **37a** show?
(b) What procedure has been carried out in **37b**?

37b

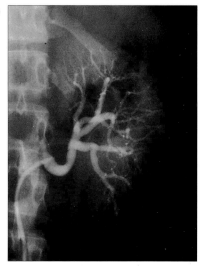

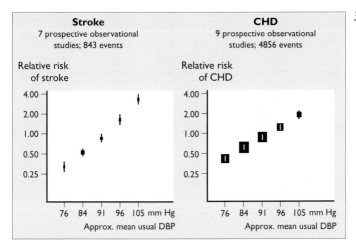

38 This figure summarises several prospective studies looking at the risk of stroke and coronary heart disease, plotted against quintiles of blood pressure. What do the sizes of the boxes indicate?

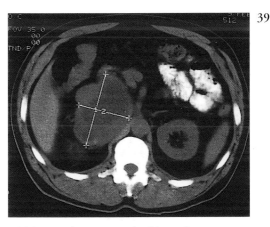

39 This 45-year-old hospital carpenter had been known to have high blood pressure for many years. He also complained of increased sweating and occasional headaches. What is the most likely diagnosis from the CT scan?

40

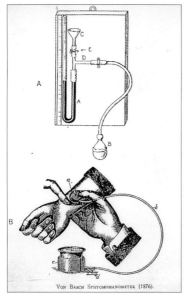

VON BASCH SPHYGMOMANOMETER (1876).

40 Von Basch, a Viennese physician, was the first to develop a practical sphygmomanometer. It was widely used to measure systolic blood pressure. Describe the principle behind this method of measuring blood pressure.

41

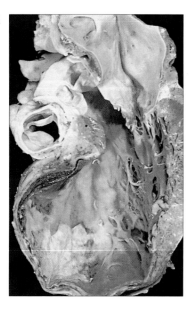

41 This 60-year-old man suffered a heart attack 6 months before his death. What complication of myocardial infarction is shown on the cross-section of his left ventricle?

42 What abnormality is shown on this renal biopsy (**42a**)? Which drug commonly used in the treatment of hypertension, may lead to this?

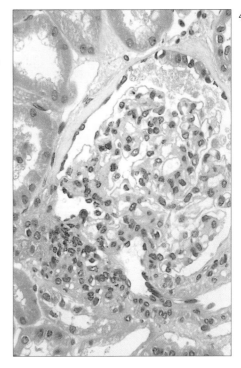

42a

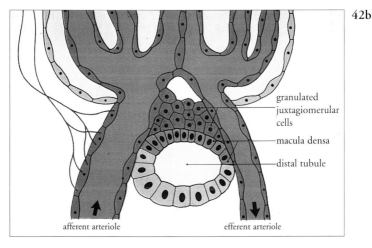

42b

granulated juxtagiomerular cells

macula densa

distal tubule

afferent arteriole

efferent arteriole

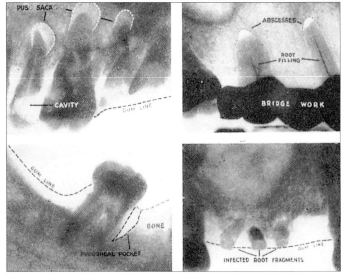

43 In the 1920s, focal infection was thought to predispose to high blood pressure, particularly infection around the teeth – *"It is not sufficient to remove teeth, obviously abscessed, but all non-vital teeth should be removed as well, as though showing extensive pyuria. Old dental cysts should be opened surgically and removed"* (George Abbot, *High Blood Pressure*, 1928). This concept is now discredited, but what common chronic infections are now thought to be associated with coronary heart disease?

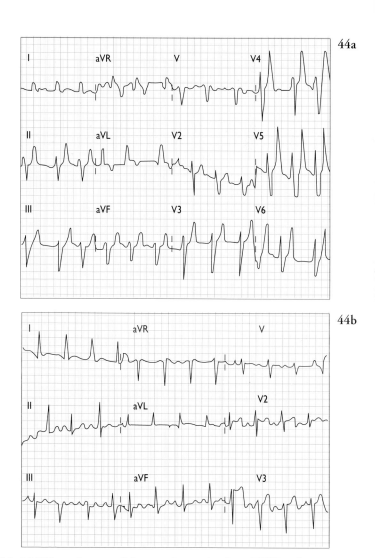

44 (a) What abnormalities are shown in these ECGs taken before and after dialysis?
(b) What combination of drugs used for treatment of high blood pressure may cause a similar but less severe problem?

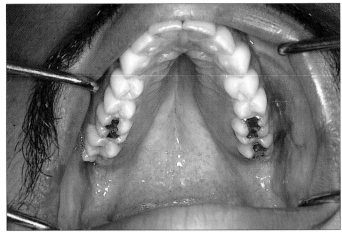

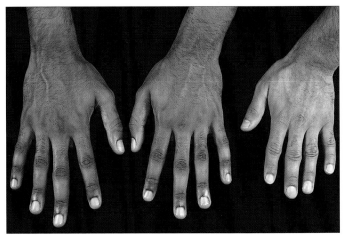

45 (a) What inherited abnormality does this 25-year-old
Afro-Caribbean man have?
(b) Is it associated with high blood pressure?

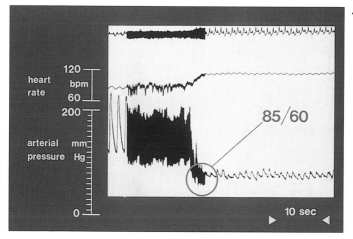

46 This illustration shows an intra-arterial blood-pressure recording in an elderly man who got up at night to pass urine. What antihypertensive drugs cause this effect?

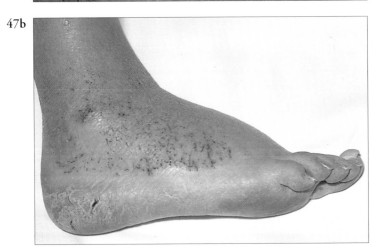

47 What is the likely cause of this rash in a middle-aged man with moderate hypertension and mild renal failure?

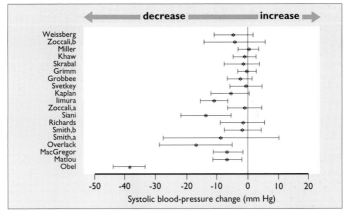

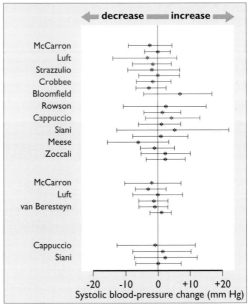

48 These illustrations summarise the results of trials on the effects of supplementation of two minerals on blood pressure. Which minerals are being studied and what are the conclusions?

49

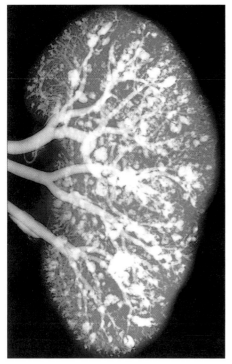

49 This illustration shows a post-mortem renal angiogram in a 55-year-old woman.
(a) What is the diagnosis?
(b) Is high blood pressure a common presenting feature of this condition?

50

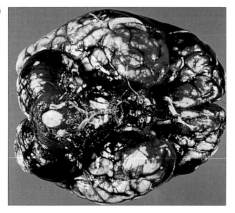

50 (a)What is the diagnosis in this post-mortem specimen?
(b)What are the likely underlying causes?

51 This 65-year-old man had severe intermittent claudication.
(a) What is shown on the angiogram?
(b) What procedure has been carried out?
(c) What are the important factors predisposing to peripheral vascular disease and what other vascular disease is likely to be present?

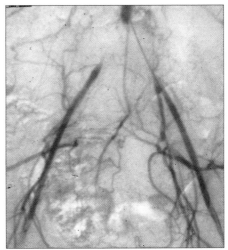
51a

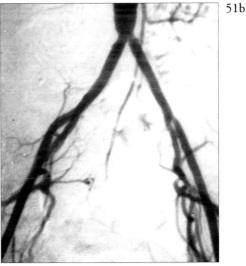
51b

52

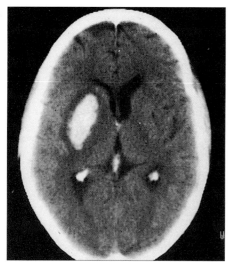

52 What does this unenhanced CT scan in a patient with high blood pressure show?

53

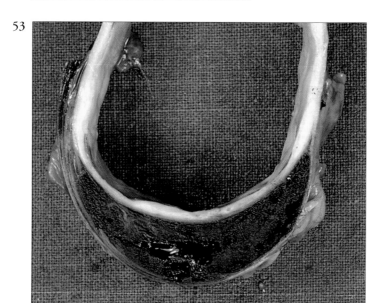

53 What does this cross-section of the aorta show?

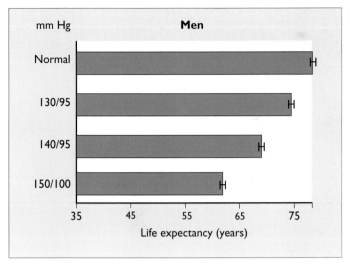

54 This figure shows life expectancy in four groups of 35-year-old men, divided according to blood pressure. The data are derived from studies by life insurance companies; the studies used a single casual measurement of the blood pressure.
(a) What is the average reduction in life expectancy in a 35-year-old man with a blood pressure of 150/100 mm Hg?
(b) Why does this data not extend to higher blood pressures?

55

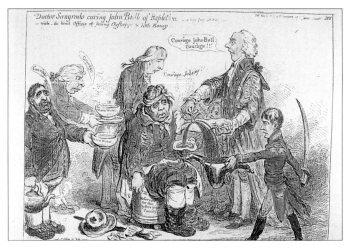

55 (a) What medical treatment is being given in this caricature?
(b) In what conditions might it have been beneficial?
(c) Would it have had any effect on high blood pressure?

56

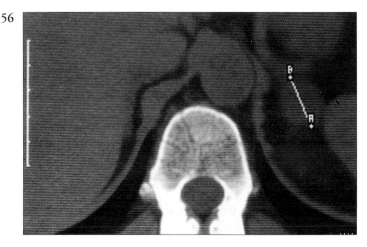

56 What are the possible diagnoses in this CT scan, which is taken at the level of the adrenal glands?

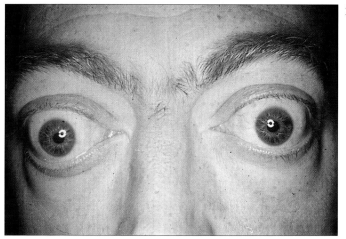

57 (a) What is the diagnosis in this 43-year-old man?
(b) Is there any relationship to high blood pressure?

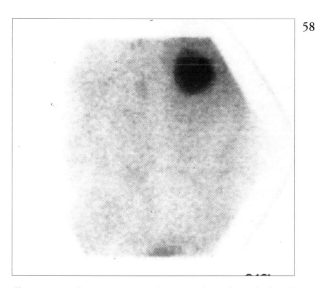

58 This illustration shows an MIBG scan taken from behind
in a 35-year-old man. What does it show?

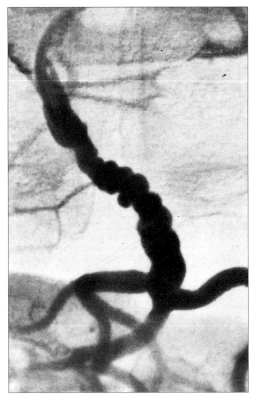

59 This is a selective renal angiogram in a 29-year-old woman with high blood pressure. What does it show?

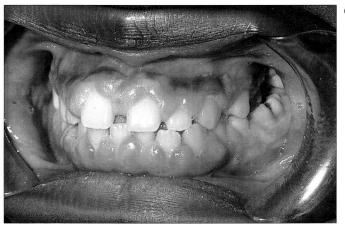

60 This man has been on long-term treatment with an antihypertensive drug. What class of drug is it likely to belong to?

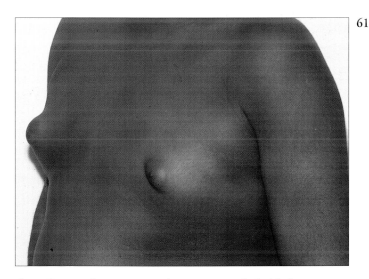

61 What antihypertensive drug is particularly likely to cause the complication seen in this patient?

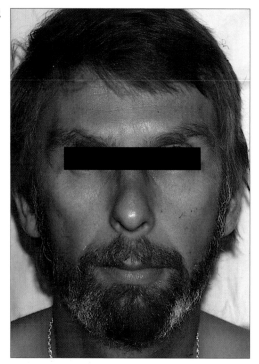

62 This 35-year-old white man, who had not been sunbathing, presented with increasing lassitude and a feeling of faintness on standing upright. What is the diagnosis?

63 What is the diagnosis in this 47-year-old man (**63b** shows his liver ultrasound)?

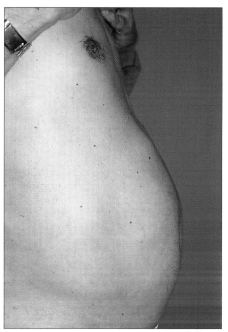
63a

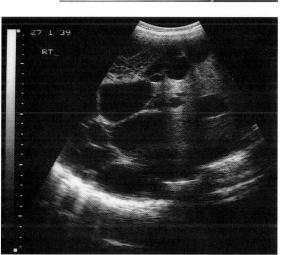
63b

64

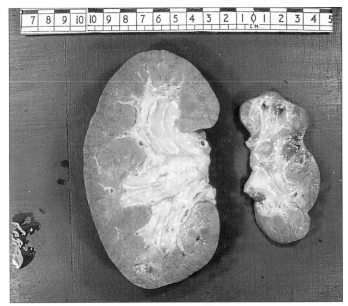

64 A 72-year-old man died from a stroke. His two kidneys are shown here in cross-section.

(a) What are the possible causes of the small size of his right kidney?

(b) Is it likely that the small size of his right kidney was causing his high blood pressure?

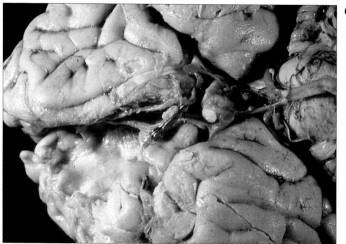

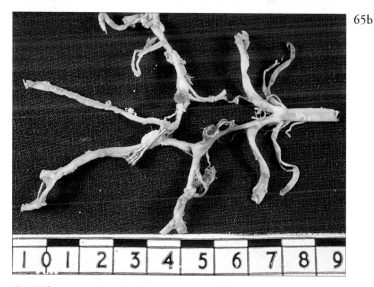

65 What procedure had been successfully carried out prior to this patient's death some years later?

66a

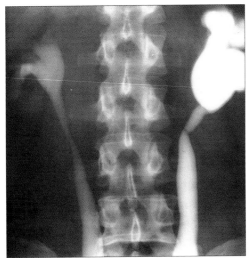

66b

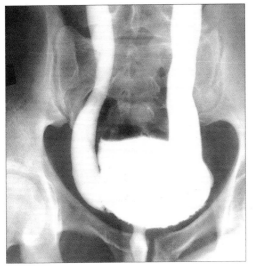

66 (a) Describe the abnormality shown on this micturating cystogram.
(b) Is this condition associated with high blood pressure?

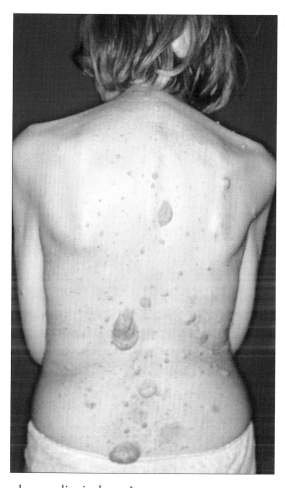

67 (a) What abnormality is shown?
(b) What is its relationship to high blood pressure?

68

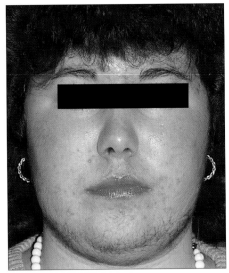

68 What syndrome does this 24-year-old woman have?

69

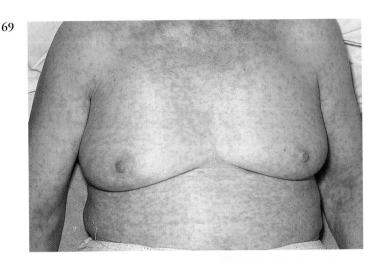

69 This 62-year-old woman was treated for high blood pressure. One week after starting drug therapy, she returned with the rash shown here. Which drugs used for the treatment of high blood pressure may cause this type of rash?

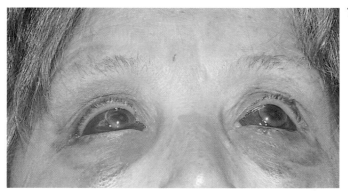

70 What abnormality is shown in this 65-year-old woman? Is there any relationship between this abnormality and blood pressure?

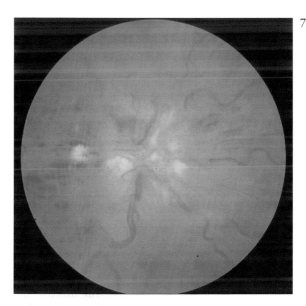

71 What is this appearance in the fundus due to? Does it occur more commonly in patients with high blood pressure?

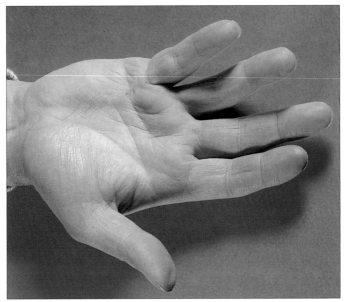

72 Is there any relationship between the abnormality shown here and high blood pressure?

73 This elderly woman presented with a painful foot and systolic hypertension. What is the likely cause of the abnormality shown in the leg? What antihypertensive drugs may make it worse?

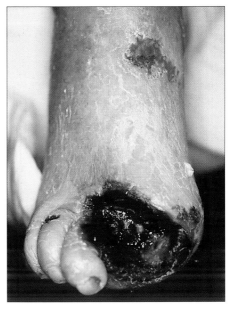

74 This man with high blood pressure and atrial fibrillation presented with progressive confusion and right-sided weakness. What does the CT scan show? How old is the abnormality? What drug is likely to have been associated with it?

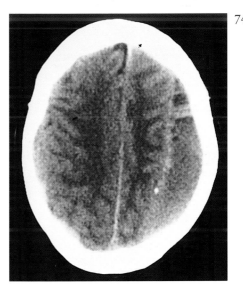

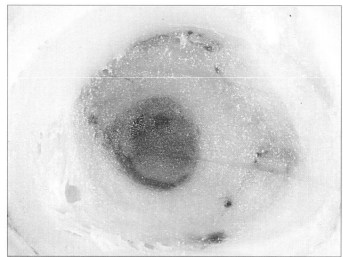

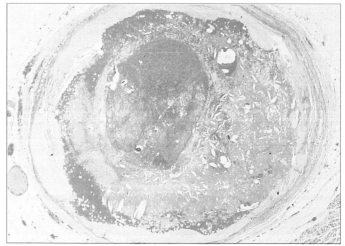

75 These illustrations show a cross-section of coronary artery obtained at post-mortem with no staining (**75a**) and the same cross-section sliced more thinly with appropriate stain (**75b**). Describe what has happened.

76 What lesion is shown in this cross-section of a brain? What symptoms might it have led to and what are the most likely predisposing causes?

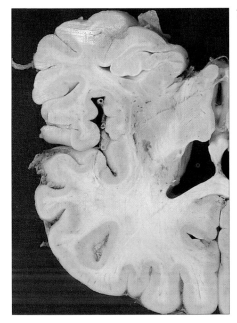

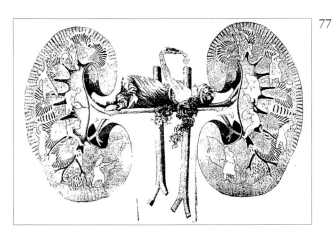

77 This illustration shows a nineteenth-century advertisement for a tonic. What sort of drug do you think it might have been, and what effect might it have had?

78

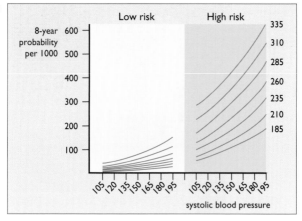

78 These graphs illustrate the probability of developing cardiovascular disease over 8 years related to systolic blood pressure (measured in mm Hg) and cholesterol levels (measured in mg/100 ml). What additional risk factors account for the very large difference in patients who are graded as low risk and those who are graded as high risk? Are any of these risk factors reversible?

79

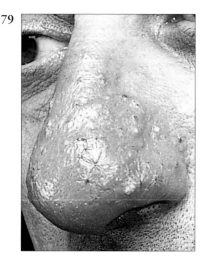

79 What is the condition shown, and what can it be due to? To what cause is it often wrongly ascribed?

80 Describe the abnormalities shown in this chest x-ray.

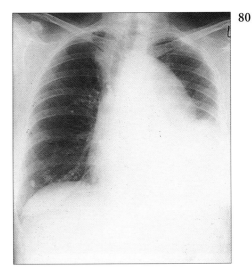

80

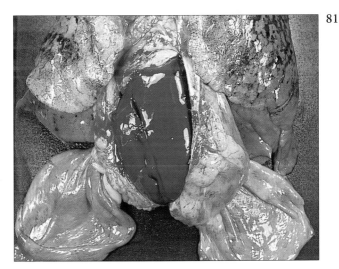

81

81 This 60-year-old man was admitted with an acute myocardial infarction.
(a) What does the post-mortem specimen show?
(b) What is the likely cause of death?

82

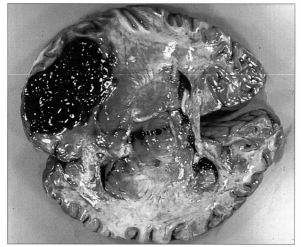

82 This man with severe hypertension died from the lesion illustrated here. What is it and where in the brain is it situated?

83

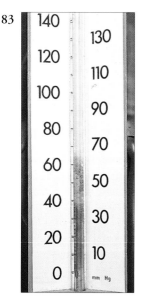

83 What is wrong with this mercury sphygmomanometer?

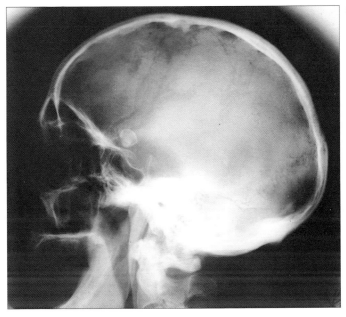

84 (a) What is shown in the skull x-ray in this 60-year-old man with high blood pressure?
(b) What might possibly be the cause of his high blood pressure?

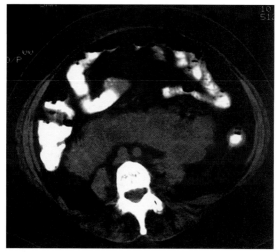

85 This illustration shows a CT scan of a young man with high blood pressure. What two abnormalities does it show and do these two often occur together?

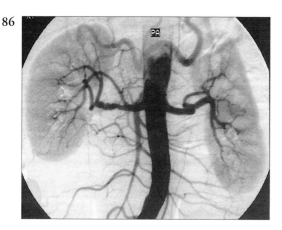

86 This illustration shows a renal angiogram of a 42-year-old woman with high blood pressure.
(a) What is the likely cause of her high blood pressure?
(b) What should be done about it?

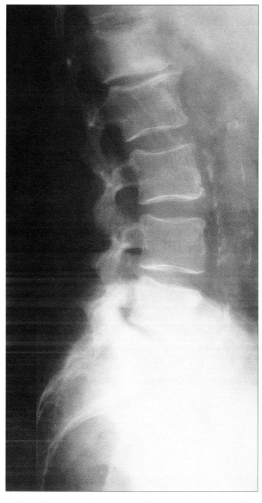

87 (a) What abnormalities are shown on this plain x-ray of the lumbar spine?
(b) Is there any relationship to high blood pressure?

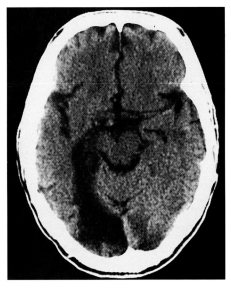

88 This illustration shows a cerebral CT scan of a 72-year-old man with treated hypertension. What abnormality is shown?

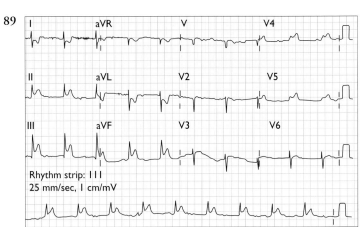

89 This illustration shows an ECG from a 54-year-old man with previous hypertension, who was admitted with severe chest pain.
(a) What does the ECG show?
(b) How would the man be treated?

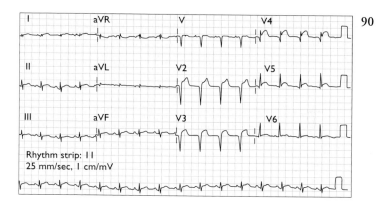

90 This is an ECG from a patient admitted with severe prolonged chest pain.
(a) What does it show?
(b) How would you treat him?

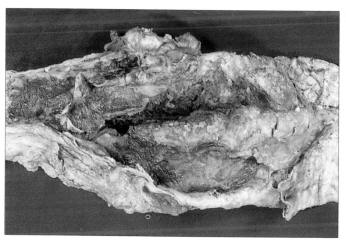

91 (a) What does this post-mortem specimen show?
(b) Is it associated with high blood pressure?

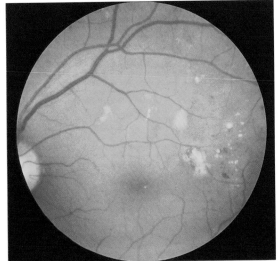

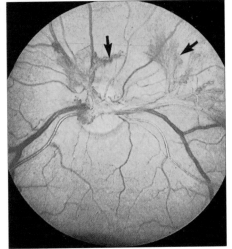

92 These two retinal photographs show typical findings.
(a) What condition underlies these two photographs?
(b) What are the relationships between these changes and those seen in hypertension?

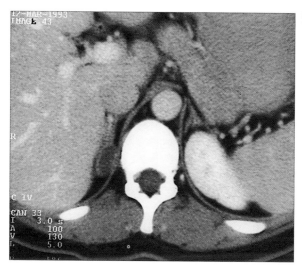

93 This illustration shows a contrast-enhanced CT scan of the abdomen.
(a) What is the diagnosis?
(b) What are the presenting features?

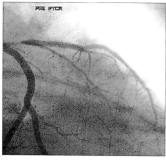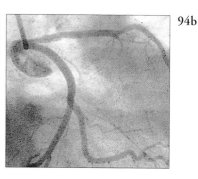

94 These two angiograms show a procedure that has been carried out.
(a) What arteries are shown?
(b) What procedure has been carried out in **94b**?

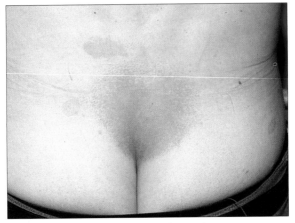

95 (a) What abnormality is shown here?
(b) What needs to be excluded in this patient?

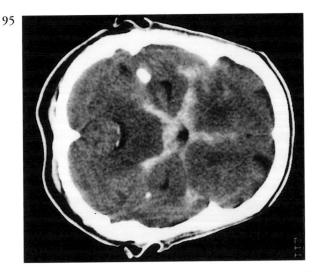

96 This 45-year-old woman had a sudden attack of severe headache and neck stiffness. What is the diagnosis as shown on the CT scan of the brain?

97 (a) What is the likely diagnosis?
(b) Is this patient likely to be thyrotoxic?

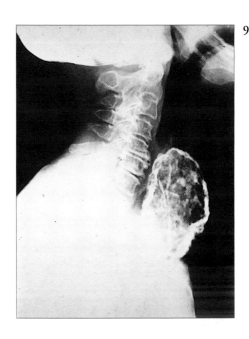

98 (a) What abnormality is shown?
(b) Can it be related to high blood pressure?

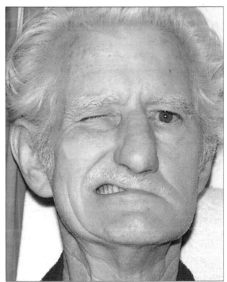

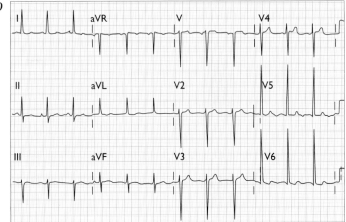

99 What changes are shown in this ECG and what is their significance?

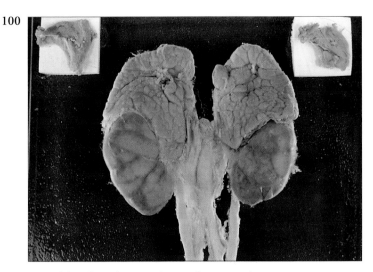

100 (a) What abnormality is shown in this post-mortem specimen from a young child?
(b) What is the likely diagnosis?

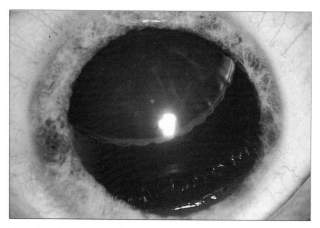

101 (a) What has happened in this eye of a 24-year-old man?
(b) What is the underlying diagnosis?

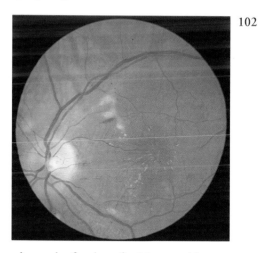

102 This illustration shows the fundus of a 32-year-old woman who presented with accelerated hypertension.
(a) Describe the changes seen.
(b) Are there any suggestions that the blood pressure may have been lowered?

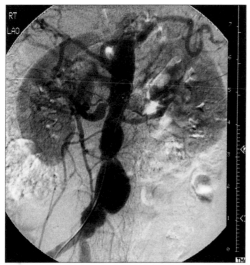

103 Describe the changes on this digital subtraction angiogram. What typical features might a patient like this have?

104 These illustrations show a CT scan (**104a**) and a post-mortem specimen of the same lesion (**104b**), but in different parts of the organ affected. What is the lesion, and which organ is it in?

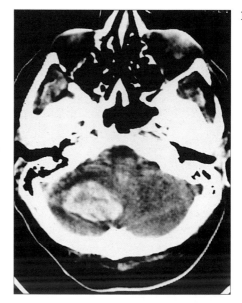

104a

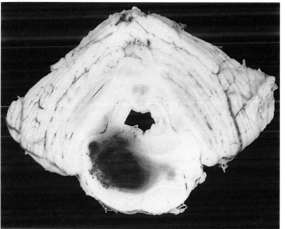

104b

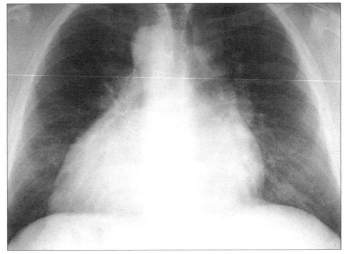

105 This illustration shows a chest x-ray of a 59-year-old man.
(a) What operation has been carried out?
(b) What abnormal features does the chest x-ray show?

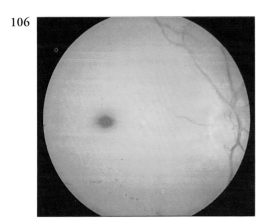

106 (a) What are these typical fundal changes due to?
(b) How would it relate to vascular disease in high blood pressure?

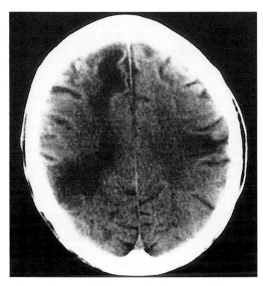

107 This illustration shows a CT scan of a hypertensive man. What lesions are shown?

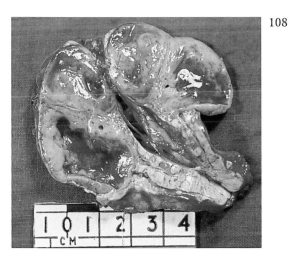

108 (a) What is the diagnosis?
(b) What are the likely symptoms?

109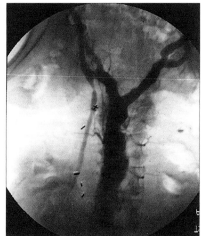

109 What abnormalities can be seen on this abdominal digital subtraction arteriogram?

110

111 This is an arteriogram in a 65-year-old man with hypertension.
(a) Which arteries are shown?
(b) What is the abnormality?
(c) What symptoms might he have?

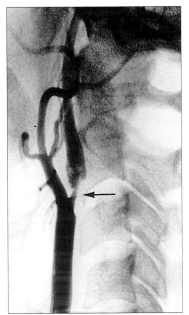

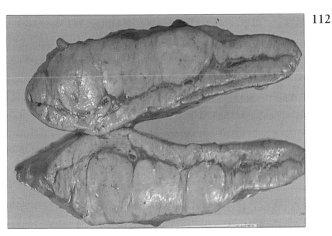

112 This illustration shows a cross-section of an adrenal gland. What is the likely diagnosis?

113

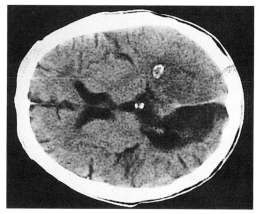

113 This 67-year-old man with treated hypertension presented with visual disturbances.
(a) What does the CT scan show?
(b) What abnormality of vision is he likely to have had?

114

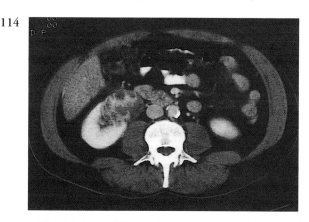

114 This is a CT scan from a 61-year-old man who had severe hypertension, and blood was found in his urine on routine testing. A renal ultrasound showed an abnormality and this was followed up by this CT scan.
(a) What does the CT scan show?
(b) What is the diagnosis?

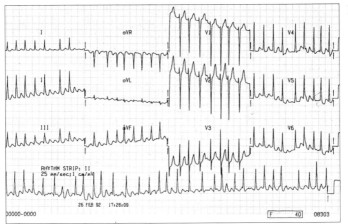

115 This is an ECG from a 55-year-old man with hypertension who had drunk a large amount of wine one evening. That night he woke up with palpitations, during which this ECG was recorded.

(a) What does the ECG show?

(b) Is the abnormality related to high blood pressure?

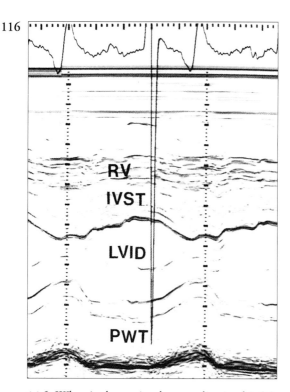

116 What is the main abnormality in this M-mode echocardiogram?

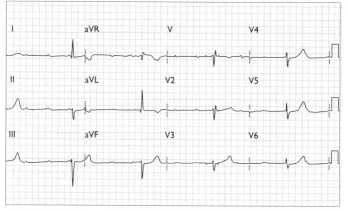

117 This ECG was recorded shortly after the patient had been treated for his hypertension.
(a) What does this ECG demonstrate?
(b) What is the antihypertensive drug most likely to cause this problem?

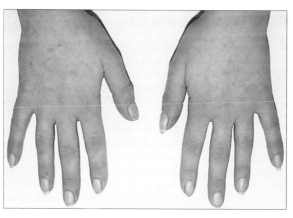

118 (a) Describe the rash shown on the hands of this young woman whose hypertension had been well controlled after one week's therapy.
(b) Which drug is the likely cause? Is this a common side effect now?

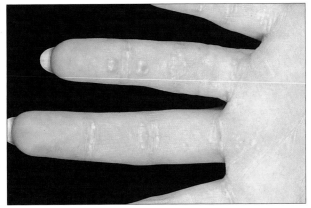

119 What is the eruption shown on the hands of this 30-year-old woman?

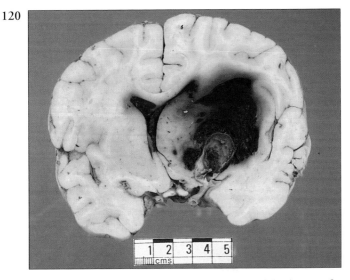

120 This is a post-mortem cross-section of the brain of a 42-year-old man who had high blood pressure. What abnormality does it demonstrate?

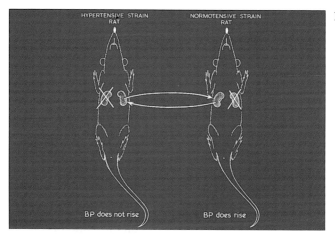

121 This diagram illustrates important experiments done in young rats with inherited hypertension and in controls. What is the potential significance of these experiments for human essential hypertension?

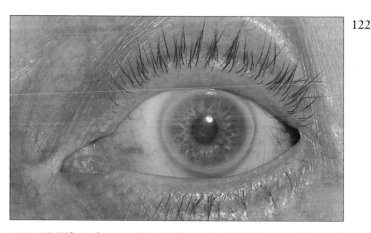

122 (a) What abnormality is shown in this 65-year-old man? (b) Is it associated with high blood pressure or with abnormal lipid disorders?

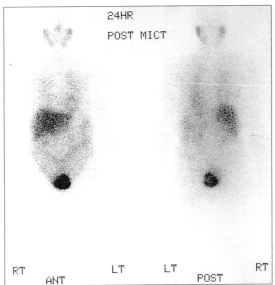

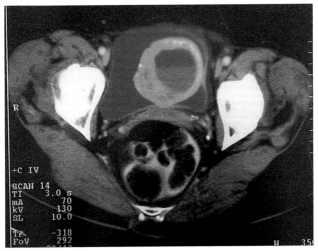

123 (a) What lesion is shown in this MIBG scan (**123a**) and CT scan at the level of the pelvis (**123b**)?

(b) What symptoms is the patient likely to have had?

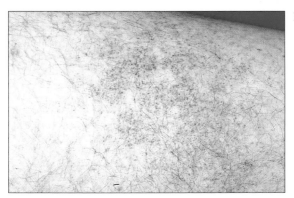

124 This rash occurred on both lower limbs of a woman treated with an antihypertensive drug. Which drug is most likely to have caused this?

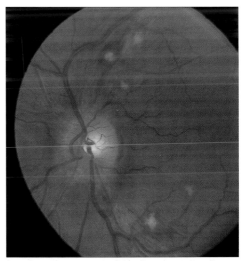

125 (a) Describe the changes seen in this photograph of a retina.
(b) What is the most likely ethnic origin of the patient?
(c) What sort of level would you expect the blood pressure to be?

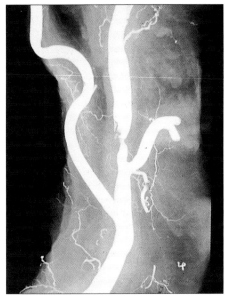

126a

126 These illustrations show a post-mortem coronary angiogram (**126a**) and a cross-section of the coronary vessel (**126b**). Describe the lesion and what has happened.

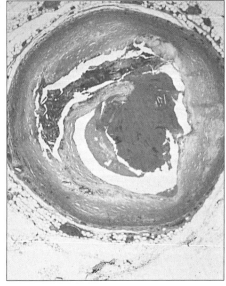

126b

ANSWERS

1   (a) The angiogram shows bilateral renal artery stenosis with an extremely tight proximal stenosis in the right artery, and a proximal and a more distal stenosis in the left artery with post-stenotic dilatation.

(b) Severe hypertension, renal impairment and heart failure.

2   (a) Stephen Hales, who carried out the first experiment to measure arterial blood pressure, on a horse, in 1733.

> "In December, I caused a mare to be tied down alive on her back. She was 14 hands high and about 14 years of age, had a fistula on her withers, was neither very lean nor yet lusty. Having laid open the left crural artery about 3" from her belly, I inserted into it a brass pipe whose bore was one sixth of an inch in diameter and to that, by means of another brass pipe which was fitly adapted to it, I fixed a glass tube of nearly the same diameter which was 9 feet in length. Then untying the ligature on the artery, the blood rose in the tube, 8 ft in length, 3" perpendicular above the level of the left ventricle of the heart."

(b) Stephen Hales subsequently measured blood pressure in many other animals and estimated from these experiments that the blood pressure in humans would represent around $7^1/_2$ feet of blood, corresponding to 176 mm Hg.

3   (a) Acute intermittent porphyria.

(b) Abdominal pain, peripheral neuropathy, hypertension.

4   (a) Angioedema.

(b) Angiotensin-converting enzyme inhibitors.

(c) If swelling affects the larynx, it may cause respiratory obstruction.

5   The figure illustrates a Chinese salt mine. The Chinese were probably the first to discover that salt preserved food. They were able to mine it by digging shafts with bamboo and extracting the salt with water. In the writings of the Yellow Emperor in approximately 2,000 B.C., it was stated "hence, if too much salt is used, the pulse hardens."

6   (a) Premature atherosclerosis.
(b) High blood pressure, smoking and increased blood cholesterol are all preventable predisposing causes.

7   (a) Gross concentric hypertrophy of the left ventricle.
(b) Hypertension. The left ventricle hypertrophies as a result of the increased workload that hypertension causes. Although this initially increases the contractile force of the left ventricle and so maintains a normal cardiac output, the hypertrophied muscle eventually outgrows its oxygen supply, causing ischaemia and cardiac failure.

8   The study illustrated compared the incidence of coronary heart disease in different countries to wine consumptions per head. The results showed that moderate alcohol consumption appears to be associated with a reduced incidence of coronary heart disease. Clearly, other factors such as diet may be important, but there is supportive evidence that wine consumption increases blood HDL cholesterol levels, and wine itself appears to contain antioxidants which may be beneficial in the prevention of coronary heart disease.

9   Rib notching, which has been caused by large collateral vessels that are secondary to coarctation of aorta.

10   Renal adenocarcinoma. About one-third of adenocarcinomas of the kidney are associated with high blood pressure, and a small number have been found to secrete renin.

11   (a) These lesions are xanthelasmas, which are composed of lipid.
(b) The patient in **11a** can just be seen to have an arcus in the left eye.
(c) The combination of xanthelasma and arcus in a patient of the young age of 25 years, as in 11a, makes it very likely that she has hypercholesterolaemia. This will require

dietary treatment and probably drug treatment. She and her first degree relatives would need to be fully investigated. Other coronary risk factors should also be looked for and treated.

Xanthelasma in older patients such as that in **11b** is very common and may not necessarily be associated with lipid abnormalities. However, they are still worth investigating.

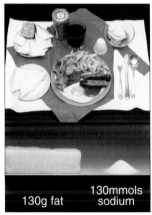 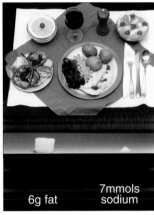

| 130g fat | 130mmols sodium | 6g fat | 7mmols sodium |

12   There is approximately 20 times more salt and fat in the top meal (**12a**; left) than in the lower meal (**12b**; right). There is also approximately three times more potassium in the healthier meal. Potassium seems to have the opposite effect to that of salt on blood pressure. Fruit and vegetables also contain other substances, e.g. vitamin C and anti-oxidants, that may prevent or delay premature vascular disease. (Note also the glass of wine in the healthy meal!)

13   (a) Henoch–Schönlein purpura.
     (b) Mesangial cell proliferation.
     (c) Hypertension is extremely common in the more severe forms of Henoch–Schönlein purpura, and it may progress to malignant hypertension. Henoch–Schönlein purpura

bears many similarities to IgA nephropathy in that they both commonly follow a respiratory tract infection and are both characterised by raised serum IgA and IgA deposition in the tissues; IgA nephropathy is also associated with severe hypertension.

14   Gross concentric hypertrophy of the left ventricle due to high blood pressure, in this case in an Afro-Caribbean man. Left ventricular hypertrophy appears to be particularly common in this group of patients, but probably reflects the severity of the hypertension. See also Question 7.

15   This is one of the first 24-hour intra-arterial ambulatory blood-pressure recordings in a normotensive subject going about his normal activities. The high-blood-pressure peaks shown at 16.00 hours and 24.00 hours are due, respectively, to a painful stimulus (a pin-prick) and coitus, with a subsequent fall in blood pressure during sleep. (Derived from Bevan, Honour & Stott. *Clin Sci* 1969: **36**: 329).

16   (a) Atrial peptides.
(b) Atrial peptides are a group of peptides that increase sodium excretion. The major circulating form is a 28 amino acid peptide which is important in the control of sodium balance and may have direct vasodilating properties. The levels of atrial peptides are raised in conditions where there is sodium and water retention, particularly in heart failure, and are also raised in many patients with high blood pressure. Drugs that inhibit the breakdown of atrial peptides have been shown to increase sodium excretion and cause a fall in blood pressure.

17   (a) Pitting oedema.
(b) Dihydropyridine calcium antagonists cause swelling of the lower legs. This is gravity dependent but is not

associated with sodium and water retention. It appears to be due to local changes in capillary haemodynamics.

(c) In some patients the oedema is transient and resolves despite continuing treatment with the drug, but in others it does not. Reducing the dose may help, but in patients with severe oedema the dihydropyridine calcium antagonist should be withdrawn.

18   The Gothenberg primary prevention study showed that subjects in whom blood pressure and blood cholesterol were both lowered showed reduced risk for premature cardiovascular disease over that of subjects in whom either blood pressure or cholesterol was reduced. This study indicates that reductions in both blood pressure and blood cholesterol have an additive effect on cardiovascular risk. These results are supported by epidemiological studies, where blood pressure and cholesterol levels have been shown to have a synergistic effect on risk. However, there have as yet been no controlled trials of lipid-lowering therapy in conjunction with blood-pressure therapy.

19   (a) The picture shows macrocytic red cells with a few target cells.

(b) The small lymphocytes give an idea of the red-cell diameter and the neutrophil is not hypersegmented. This indicates that the patient is probably drinking large amounts of alcohol, has liver disease or hypothyroidism. High alcohol intake can cause resistant hypertension. Surreptitious high alcohol intake may be revealed by measurement of mean corpuscular volume or liver enzymes.

20   The scan shows a large mass above, or in continuation with, the left kidney. Possible diagnoses would include hypernephroma of the left kidney, phaeochromocytoma, and adrenal carcinoma, either primary or secondary. This patient had a primary adrenal carcinoma with associated hypertension. Adrenal carcinoma is an extremely rare cause of hypertension.

21 This is the second Veterans Administration Trial (1970), conducted in men with diastolic pressures between 90 and 114 mm Hg. The illustration shows the clear effect of treatment in reducing events such as strokes, heart failure, progression of renal disease and, though non-significantly, heart attacks. Sub-group analysis shows that the main benefits were largely confined to patients with diastolic pressures between 105 and 114 mm Hg.

22 This method of blood-pressure measurement depended on volume displacement with every pulse beat. If four fingers were used there was a greater volume displacement and the blood-pressure recordings were more accurate.

23 Tophaceous gout, which can be aggravated by treatment with diuretics.

24 (a) There is diffuse enlargement of the heart.
(b) Causes include pericardial effusion, ischaemic heart disease, cardiomyopathy and hypertension. In this patient the enlargement of the heart was due to left ventricular hypertrophy caused by severe hypertension.

25 The venom of the Brazilian arrowhead viper (*Bothrops jararaca*) contains many peptides, several of which were shown in 1965 to potentiate the effect of bradykinin. These were further isolated into a pure nonapeptide, SQ20881 (teprotide), which is a specific inhibitor of angiotensin-converting enzyme (ACE), the enzyme responsible for conversion of angiotensin I to angiotensin II. This led to the development of orally active ACE inhibitors, the first of which was 'Captopril'.

26 (a) A large phaeochromocytoma.
(b) The tumour shows multiple haemorrhagic areas.
(c) Phaeochromocytomas commonly cause headache, sweating, palpitations and hypertension due to sudden release of large amounts of catecholamines. This patient was unusual in that he had only mild hypertension with

very few symptoms indicative of phaeochromocytoma. Fortunately, he was diagnosed on routine screening for urinary metabolites of noradrenaline and adrenaline.

27   Intracerebral haemorrhage with medial displacement, probably due to severe hypertension.

28   Gross papilloedema, flame-shaped haemorrhages and exudates. This is the typical fundal appearance of malignant or accelerated hypertension. This patient's blood pressure was extremely high at 246/144 mm Hg, and there were symptoms of left ventricular failure. Creatinine was 20 μmol/l. With a gradual reduction in blood pressure over a few days, the heart failure disappeared and renal function returned towards normal.

29   This is the typical facies of a patient on long-term minoxidil treatment. The patient exhibits coarsening of his facial features and increased hair growth, particularly coming down from the hairline towards the eyes. Minoxidil is a very effective vasodilator, once routinely used to control blood pressure. However, due to the gross sodium and water retention it causes, requiring large doses of diuretics, and the associated severe hair growth, it is now infrequently used.

30   A typical golden-yellow adrenal adenoma, which causes primary aldosteronism. Presenting features include low plasma potassium, high plasma sodium and severe hypertension. Diagnosis can be confirmed by a finding of low plasma renin activity, high aldosterone and by CT scanning.

31   (a) Accelerated/malignant hypertension.
(b) There is gross narrowing of the lumen of the arteriole with intimal proliferation. The consequent reduction in renal blood flow to the glomerulus activates the renin-angiotensin system. If there are sufficient numbers of arterioles narrowed, this will cause renal failure. In some

cases this renal failure is reversible with careful control of blood pressure.

32 (a) Subdural haematoma.
    (b) Head injury, high alcohol intake, increasing age and high blood pressure. In many the high blood pressure may be due to high alcohol intake.
    (c) Headache and confusion.

33 (a) Enlarged polycystic kidney with the renal parenchyma almost entirely replaced by numerous thin-walled cysts.
    (b) High blood pressure very commonly develops before the onset of renal failure. Patients with polycystic kidneys are more likely to develop strokes, partly because of high blood pressure and partly because of an increased incidence of berry aneurysms in the cerebral circulation. Careful control of the raised blood pressure will reduce strokes and may slow the rate of decline of renal function.

34 (a) Acromegaly.
    (b) Acromegalic patients commonly have high blood pressure and left ventricular hypertrophy.

35 (a) Horseshoe kidney.
    (b) Urinary tract infection, renal calculi and urinary obstruction. Hypertension is not usually a feature.

36 (a) Scleroderma/systemic sclerosis. There is characteristic thickening and tightening of the skin around the fingers.
    (b) Blood pressure is usually normal but becomes raised when the kidneys are involved, often presenting with fulminant accelerated hypertension and renal failure. The renal failure may possibly be prevented by early treatment of high blood pressure.

37 (a) Severe renal artery stenosis due to a fibrous band.
    (b) Balloon angioplasty has been carried out, with very successful dilatation of the renal artery. The patient became normotensive and remained so on follow-up.

38   The sizes of the boxes indicate the number of people affected by coronary heart disease compared to strokes. Patients are far more likely to develop coronary heart disease than stroke and it is a more common cause of death in Western countries.

39   This is a large phaeochromocytoma. In many patients, the larger the phaeochromocytoma, the fewer symptoms it causes. The tumour was successfully removed over 5 years ago with no recurrence. Blood pressure fell to normal.

40   Dr Von Basch first used his machine in 1876. It utilised a pelote, connected as shown to a reservoir and mercury sphygmomanometer. An artery that lies directly on the bone, such as the temporal artery or the radial artery, is selected and pressure is exerted on it with the membrane of the pelote. The pressure thus exerted on the artery is transmitted through the water-filled system to the mercury-filled manometer. The pulse is simultaneously felt with a finger, just beyond the point of compression. The manometer is read at the moment when the pulse disappears as the pressure is increased and again at the moment it first returns as the pressure is decreased. The mercury sphygmomanometer was rather cumbersome, and Von Basch went on to develop a metal manometer, which was more portable. Modern sphygmomanometers still use this principle of measurement but with a cuff and auscultation. However, palpation of the radial or brachial artery should still be used for measurement of systolic pressure before auscultation in order to avoid a falsely low systolic pressure reading due to a silent gap in the Korotkov sounds.

41   There is a large ventricular aneurysm. This is a late complication of myocardial infarction. Patients usually present with heart failure, arrhythmias or emboli. There is usually a persistent ST segment on ECG. Sometimes there is a visible bulge on the chest x-ray. Diagnosis is confirmed by 2-D echocardiography.

42 This slide shows gross juxtaglomerular hyperplasia due to prolonged treatment with frusemide. It is important to remember that diuretics stimulate the renin-angiotensin system and in the long term cause juxtaglomerular hyperplasia. The increased release of renin may continue for some time after the diuretic has been withdrawn.

43 Infection with either *Helicobacter pylori* or *Chlamydia pneumoniae* are now thought to be associated with coronary heart disease.

44 (a) This patient, who was on intermittent haemodialysis, had missed one of his routine dialyses. Potassium before dialysis was 9.5 mmol/l; after dialysis the potassium fell to 3.4 mmol/l. In the pre-dialysis ECG, characteristic changes of high potassium with peak T waves are seen.
(b) Small increases in plasma potassium in patients with hypertension may occur with converting enzyme inhibitors and distally acting diuretics. Major increases in plasma potassium are rare, however, though they can occur when ACE inhibitors are used in patients in acute renal failure or in patients who are rejecting a renal transplant.

45 (a) These illustrations show arachnodactyly and a high arched palate, both of which are characteristic of Marfan's syndrome.
(b) Marfan's syndrome is a connective tissue disorder which gives rise to mitral valve prolapse and regurgitation, aortic incompetence, aortic dilatation and dissection, as well as lens dislocation. To prevent aortic dissection it is vital that very good control of the blood pressure is maintained throughout life. It is therefore important that these patients have regular checks on their blood pressure and are treated with drugs at blood-

pressure levels where treatment is not usually indicated in patients with essential hypertension.

46 This patient was on a post-adrenergic blocking drug, debrisoquine. Note that the supine blood pressure is uncontrolled, but when he stands up there is profound postural hypotension. This phenomenon is almost invariably seen with these drugs (when the blood pressure is measured carefully enough), and drugs such as debrisoquine, guanethidine, and bethanidine should now not be used in the treatment of high blood pressure.

47 This shows the typical features of an underlying vasculitis. The vasculitic disorders include a wide range of conditions, including polyarteritis nodosa. This man had polyarteritis nodosa with severe hypertension and moderate renal impairment.

48 **48a** shows a summary of the studies looking at the effect of potassium chloride supplementation on blood pressure before the potassium was given, or during the placebo phase. It can be seen that the higher the blood pressure, the greater the effect of potassium supplementation and overall there was a significant fall in blood pressure.
48b shows the studies of effects of calcium supplementation on blood pressure. It can be seen overall that there is no effect of calcium supplementation on blood pressure whether in the high or normal range.

49 (a) The post-mortem arteriogram shows multiple aneurysms and it is very suggestive of polyarteritis nodosa.
(b) High blood pressure is an extremely common presenting feature of polyarteritis nodosa, as well as skin rash (see **47a**) and renal impairment. This patient in fact presented with severe hypertension and renal impairment.

50 (a) Subarachnoid haemorrhage.
(b) There is an increased frequency of subarachnoid haemorrhage in patients with polycystic kidney disease who not only may have raised blood pressure, but seem also to have an increased incidence of cerebral aneurysms. High blood pressure itself predisposes to subarachnoid haemorrhage, both pre-existing Berry aneurysms, as well as in the Charcot-Bouchard aneurysms.

51 (a) Digital subtraction angiography shows severe stenosis of both iliac arteries at the junction with the aorta.
(b) Balloon angioplasty has been carried out.
(c) Peripheral vascular disease is predisposed to by cigarette smoking, high blood pressure, and high cholesterol levels, as well as by diabetes. The vascular disease is not confined to the limbs and it is extremely common to find that these patients have renal artery stenosis, cerebrovascular atheroma, particularly in the carotid arteries, and coronary artery disease.

52 This 55-year-old man had severe hypertension, which was presumably the direct cause of his subarachnoid haemorrhage. Further investigation did not reveal any underlying cerebral aneurysm.

53 Aortic dissection. There is clotted blood in the channel that has been created by the dissection, and the aorta is seen above it. Aortic dissection is much more common in patients with high blood pressure.

54 (a) These life insurance studies found that a man of 35 who had a single casual measurement of blood pressure of 150/100 mm Hg had on average a reduction in life expectancy of $16^1/_2$ years. This emphasises the very important predictive role of even mild elevations in blood pressure on premature mortality over a long period of time. It contrasts with the trials of treatment which have been limited to only a short time span and in younger subjects with mild hypertension, who do not show much evidence of benefit. Unfortunately, studies over a longer period of time have not yet been carried out and, therefore, the benefits of treatment in younger patients with mild hypertension are not so clearcut.

(b) Where blood pressure was found to exceed 150/100 mm Hg, insurance was not issued and there was no follow-up on these subjects. Therefore, no data was collected. It was, of course, already known that patients with a blood pressure over 150/100 mm Hg died earlier than others.

55 (a) The subject is being bled and purged. This was common therapy in the 18th and early 19th century. Many famous people (and countless others) were killed by this treatment, including Charles II of England and Louis XIV of France.

(b) Purging caused severe diarrhoea with loss of sodium and water. In conjunction with removal of blood, this would cause a large reduction in intravascular fluid volume. This treatment, therefore, would have been good therapy for left ventricular failure and congestive heart failure, at least temporarily.

(c) It would also have produced a transient reduction in blood pressure!

56 There is a mass in the left adrenal gland. Differential diagnoses include phaeochromocytoma, a non-functioning adenoma, or an aldosterone-producing adenoma. This woman presented with a plasma potassium of 1.8 mmol/l and a plasma sodium of 145 mmol/l, and she had severe hypertension. She was subsequently found to have low renin and high aldosterone. The adrenal adenoma was removed and her blood pressure returned to normal.

57 (a) This man has marked thyrotoxic eye disease, which is commonly associated with thyrotoxicosis.
(b) Thyrotoxicosis causes activation of the sympathetic nervous system and widening of the pulse pressure; there is also often an increase in heart rate. Blood pressure in this man was slightly raised at 154/90 mm Hg. With control of his thyrotoxicosis, his blood pressure fell into the normal range.

58 A large right adrenal phaeochromocytoma.

59 Typical appearances of fibromuscular hyperplasia. Although there does not seem to be any obviously gross narrowing of the artery, this can be very deceptive on arteriograms since there may well be a web across the artery, causing significant obstruction in these patients. If there is a reduction in blood flow to the kidney, angioplasty is usually remarkably successful.

60 There is gingival hyperplasia, which is occasionally associated with the use of the dihydropyridine calcium antagonists. It can also occur with phenytoin treatment for epilepsy.

61 Spironolactone, particularly in high doses used for the treatment of primary aldosteronism, may cause gynaecomastia. Reserpine was also occasionally associated with gynaecomastia. Withdrawal of spironolactone results in the disappearance of the gynaecomastia.

62 Addison's disease. This patient has developed gross pigmentation secondary to the failure of the adrenal glands. His blood pressure on presentation showed a supine value of 110/65 mm Hg; on standing it fell to 80 mm Hg systolic with an unrecordable diastolic. Plasma sodium was low, plasma renin was extremely high, with no measurable aldosterone. The failure of the adrenal cortex results in loss of cortisol secretion.

However, most of the symptoms of Addison's disease are due to sodium and water loss secondary to lack of aldosterone. It is important when treating these patients not only to replace the cortisol, but also to replace the mineralocorticoids with fludrocortisone. The dose of fludrocortisone should be adjusted according to the patient's plasma potassium, weight, blood pressure, and, ideally, measurement of plasma renin activity.

63 (a) He has swelling of the abdomen. Ultrasound confirmed this to be due to multiple renal cysts. This patient has bilateral polycystic kidney disease with severe hypertension and large cysts in his liver.

64 (a) The small size of the kidney may have several causes, including congenital maldevelopment, reflux nephropathy, or renal artery stenosis. In this particular man, the renal artery was small but not narrowed and there was no evidence of reflux.

(b) In the past, many patients have had small kidneys such as this removed, with little justification. At the very least, renal vein renin levels with determinations made above and below the renal veins should be done before removing these kidneys. Unless there is clear evidence that renin secretion is much higher on the side of the small kidney, removal is not justified, as the small kidney is unlikely to be causing high blood pressure.

65 A clip can be seen on a berry aneurysm on the circle of Willis. This is more clearly seen when the circle of Willis is dissected out (**65b**). There is also atrophy of the frontal lobe.

66 (a) The micturating cystogram shows gross reflux in both ureters from the bladder to the kidney. There is dilatation of the pelvis on the left side and calyceal dilatation.

(b) Reflux nephropathy is commonly associated with high blood pressure, particularly when there is associated renal impairment.

67   (a) Pedunculated neurofibromatosis.
(b) This condition is associated with phaeochromocytoma. Anyone with this condition should have his or her blood pressure and catecholamine excretion measured in order to exclude a phaeochromocytoma.

68   This woman shows the typical signs of excess cortisol – hirsutism, acne, florid appearance, and increased fat deposition in the face. The most common cause of this is treatment with steroids, but in this woman it was found to be due to oversecretion of cortisol. Blood pressure was slightly raised and fell within the normal range when her Cushing's syndrome was treated.

69   This is a typical maculopapular drug rash. All of the drugs used for the treatment of hypertension may cause this type of rash. This rash was due to a thiazide diuretic; when the drug was stopped, the rash resolved.

70   Bilateral conjunctival haemorrhage. In this particular woman it was due to prolonged coughing and vomiting. Contrary to common belief, it is not related to high blood pressure.

71   The fundus shows the typical changes of retinal vein occlusion – the classic 'sunset' appearance and engorgement of the veins. Note the presence of normal-looking arterioles. It is not clear whether retinal vein occlusion is more common in patients with high blood pressure, but it is an important differential diagnosis from papilloedema with haemorrhages and exudates.

72 The abnormality shown is Dupuytren's contracture. The majority of cases are idiopathic, but there is an increased incidence in patients with chronic liver disease and cirrhosis secondary to excess alcohol, which, in itself, may cause high blood pressure. Certain drugs such as phenytoin are also associated with Dupuytren's contracture and high blood pressure.

73 The gangrene of the foot is most likely to be secondary to diabetes mellitus and severe vascular disease. Diabetics commonly develop high blood pressure and careful treatment may prevent the complications, particularly by slowing down the progression of the renal disease. Beta-blockers reduce peripheral blood flow and should not be used in patients with peripheral vascular disease.

74 There is a large left subdural haematoma with the same density as surrounding tissue, suggesting that it is recent. There was no history of injury and it is likely that the warfarin that he was taking for his atrial fibrillation was the cause.

75 There is the typical appearance of a large plaque in the coronary artery, which has ruptured. A thrombus has occluded the remaining space, thereby causing acute myocardial infarction. High blood pressure is a major risk factor for coronary artery disease.

76 There is a small infarct in the internal capsule. This will cause a complete hemiparesis. The most likely predisposing cause is hypertension. This figure illustrates how a small lesion in a critical area of the brain can have devastating effects.

77 The advertisement is for a uricosuric, presumably one based on aspirin. The use of these tonics was based on the

idea that the tablet will clean and flush out the kidneys. Plasma uric acid levels are raised in patients with hypertension, but there is no evidence, as yet, that reducing uric acid levels in patients who do not have gout is of any benefit.

78 The low-risk patients do not have glucose intolerance, do not smoke, and have no evidence of left ventricular hypertrophy on ECG, whereas the high-risk patients have glucose intolerance, smoke cigarettes, and have left ventricular hypertrophy on ECG. It is of overwhelming importance that patients with hypertension stop smoking. Careful treatment and control of the blood pressure will cause regression of left ventricular hypertrophy; loss of weight by restriction of calorie intake may cause improvements in glucose intolerance; however, whether this reduces the risk of vascular disease is not clear at present.

79 A rhinophyma. This is a disorder of middle-aged men which is usually associated with rosacea, and the enlargement of the nose is produced by hyperplasia of the sebaceous glands. It is commonly thought to be related to excessive alcohol intake, for which there is very little evidence, and many people think that there is a relationship with high blood pressure, though again there is no evidence for this.

80 There is a great increase in the width of the mediastinum at the level of the aortic arch, with loss of definition of the aortic outline and deviation of the trachea to the right. There is also filling in of the left costophrenic angle. An intravenous digital subtraction angiogram showed aortic dissection in the ascending and descending aorta.

81 (a) This man had a large anterior myocardial infarction. (b) The heart ruptured causing cardiac tamponade. Blood surrounding the heart can be seen.

82 There is a large cerebral haemorrhage in the frontal lobe.

83 The glass tube in the mercury sphygmomanometer is coated with dirt and oxides of mercury, obscuring the column. The mercury column is at zero. Mercury sphygmomanometers should be regularly serviced and the service should include cleaning the glass tube – otherwise inaccurate measurements of blood pressure may result.

84 (a) A calcified aneurysm. (b) This man has polycystic kidney disease.

85 The CT scan of the abdomen shows a horse-shoe kidney with multiple cysts, i.e. polycystic kidney disease. This combination is a rare finding.

86 (a) This digital subtraction renal arteriogram shows the typical appearances of fibromuscular hyperplasia in the distal part of the main right renal artery. Note the corkscrew appearance. The left renal artery, as far as it can be seen, looks normal. There does not appear to be any severe narrowing of the right renal artery, but this may be deceptive on arteriograms as a web across the renal artery could cause obstruction. (b) The patient had an angioplasty, and her blood pressure, at least over the first year of follow-up, fell considerably to the point that she no longer needed to be on antihypertensive drugs.

87 (a) The aorta is calcified but it can be seen to be of normal dimensions.

(b) It is very common for arteries, particularly the aorta, to become calcified in older subjects, and there does not seem to be any definite relationship to vascular disease. Even so, stiffening of the arteries, of which this is a more advanced form, may be part of the mechanism of the elevated systolic pressure that can occur in old age.

88 The CT scan shows a large occipital infarct.

89 (a) The ECG shows acute ST elevation in leads 2, 3 and AVF, demonstrating an acute inferior myocardial infarction. In addition there are reciprocal changes in the lateral leads.
(b) He was treated with diamorphine, streptokinase and aspirin.

90 (a) There is extensive anterior ST elevation with Q waves across the chest leads with reciprocal inferior changes.
(b) Diamorphine should be given for pain relief, and streptokinase and aspirin for their thrombolytic action.

91 (a) This is an abdominal aneurysm that has burst.
(b) Abdominal aneurysms are much more common in patients with high blood pressure and are more likely to rupture in these patients.

92 (a) **92a** shows typical background diabetic retinopathy – hard exudates consisting of lipid deposits, and deep haemorrhages with dot-and-blot appearance. **92b** shows the typical appearances of severe proliferative diabetic retinopathy. Fronds of new vessels can be seen emerging from the disc and elsewhere.
(b) In **92a** the macula is not involved and the vessels are completely normal. This differentiates it from hypertensive changes where the vessels will be abnormal.

The changes in **92b** are particularly seen in diabetics who have renal impairment and hypertension.

93   (a) This CT scan shows a low density, non-enhancing tumour in the posterior limb of the right adrenal gland, with a thin capsule and dimensions 2cm × 1cm. The appearances are typical of an adrenal adenoma secreting aldosterone.

(b) This 33-year-old woman presented with blood pressure of 180/110 mm Hg, potassium of 2.9 mmol/l, plasma sodium of 144 mmol/l, bicarbonate 31 mmol/l. Subsequent removal of the adenoma was successful, blood pressure fell to normal, and electrolytes returned to normal values.

94   (a) The coronary angiogram (**94a**) shows a severe stenosis of the origin of the left anterior descending coronary artery.

(b) In **94b**, a successful angioplasty has been carried out.

95   (a) This patient has café-au-lait spots.

(b) These are associated with phaeochromocytoma, although this particular patient had normal blood pressure and normal 24-hour excretion of catecholamine metabolites.

96   Subarachnoid haemorrhage can be secondary to intracerebral haemorrhage, or primary due to an aneurysm of the circle of Willis, arteriovenous malformation, bleeding tumour or a haemorrhagic diathesis. There is a well known association between adult polycystic kidney disease and aneurysms of the circle of Willis.

97   (a) The x-ray shows a long-standing calcified, multi-nodular goitre.

(b) In general, these patients are euthyroid. In this particular patient there was mild thyrotoxicosis and mildly raised blood pressure.

98 (a) This man has a left facial palsy.
(b) Accelerated hypertension is sometimes associated with facial palsies. The reason for this is not clear.

99 The ECG shows changes compatible with severe left ventricular hypertrophy. It shows that the sum of the S wave in V2 and the R wave in V6 is greater than 35 mm, and in lead V6 there is ST depression compatible with 'LV strain'.

100 (a) There is gross enlargement of both adrenal glands. (The inset shows the normal size of the adrenal glands for a child of this age.)
(b) This child had 11-beta-hydroxylase deficiency; lack of this enzyme prevents the hydroxylation of 11-deoxycortisol, leading to low cortisol levels. The defect also prevents the conversion of 11-deoxycorticosterone to corticosterone and aldosterone. The low levels of cortisol induce very high levels of ACTH, which results in very high 11-deoxycorticosterone levels, thereby leading to virilisation, hypertension, and hypokalaemia. Treatment is with glucocorticoids.

101 (a) The lens has been 'subluxed' (dislocated). The serrated edge of the lens can be clearly seen and this is where it is normally attached.
(b) This strongly suggests that the patient has Marfan's syndrome. Good control of blood pressure may possibly prevent aortic dissection and rupture (another complication of Marfan's syndrome), but there is no evidence that control of blood pressure reduces the problem of lens subluxation.

102 (a) This fundus demonstrates the typical features of accelerated hypertension, with cotton wool spots, and oedema of the macular with striae, hard exudates, and the beginnings of a macular star. There are a few flame-shaped haemorrhages.
(b) There is no papilloedema but there are striae around the disc, suggesting that there has been swelling of the optic disc which has resolved. Indeed, this was the situation, as her blood pressure had been reduced before this photograph was taken. Notice also the arteriovenous nipping.

103 The renal angiogram shows severe atheromatous disease with markedly diseased iliac vessels and aorta with a large aortic aneurysm. There is narrowing of both renal arteries at the origin, more marked on the right side with probable post-stenotic dilatation. This patient was a heavy cigarette smoker, and had a cholesterol of 9.3 mmol/l. Blood pressure was 180/110 mm Hg when first seen. Plasma creatinine was 210 µmol/l. She was 65 years old and originally presented with intermittent claudication.

104 The CT scan and the post-mortem specimen both show a large cerebellar haemorrhage.

105 (a) This man has had coronary artery surgery.
(b) The sternum has been split and there are clips on the left side of the border of the heart, where the coronary bypass has been inserted. The heart is enlarged. There is prominence of the veins with pulmonary venous congestion.

106 (a) This shows the typical appearances of central retinal artery occlusion. The arteries are very thin or absent, and

there is fragmented blood in those that are visible. The retina is swollen with a cherry-red spot at the fovea.

(b) These changes are nearly always associated with embolisation, particularly cholesterol emboli (for instance from carotid artery disease, which is commonly associated with high blood pressure).

107 There are multiple large cerebral infarcts. Although this may be due to thrombosis, it is important to exclude multiple emboli.

108 (a) This is a cross-section of an adrenal gland containing a phaeochromocytoma in a young man. The remnants of the adrenal gland can still be seen.

(b) This patient had severe hypertension in the accelerated phase, with sweating, headaches, and palpitations.

109 There is severe vascular disease of the iliac vessels and aorta, and there are no native renal arteries visible. There is a saphenous vein graft coming from the iliac vessel up to the left kidney. There is a stenosis in the vein graft shortly after the origin from the iliac vessel. Metal clips can also be seen. This patient presented with severe heart failure for which there was no obvious cause. A renal angiogram showed that the right renal artery was blocked and there was a very tight stenosis of the left renal artery. Following renal bypass surgery the patient had a massive sodium and water diuresis and her heart failure resolved. A year subsequently she developed stenosis as shown on the x-ray here. This was successfully angioplastied and she remains well.

110 The aortic arch is seen in cross-section above the heart. The black area within the aortic arch represents flowing blood. It can be seen that there is dissection within the

aortic aneurysm. To the right and above this is an area that is grayer and a whitish area. These represent either clot or slow-flowing blood. Below the aorta the left ventricle can clearly be seen in cross-section.

111 (a) This is a carotid angiogram.
(b) It shows severe narrowing of the internal carotid at its origin with a probable post-stenotic dilatation.
(c) This man was suffering from transient ischaemic attacks.

112 The adrenal gland is diffusely enlarged. The patient had Cushing's disease secondary to a pituitary adenoma, with bilateral enlargement of both adrenal glands.

113 (a) The CT scan shows a large occipital infarct.
(b) He had homonymous hemianopia.

114 (a) The CT scan shows a large, solid mass arising from the right kidney.
(b) These appearances are typical of adenocarcinoma of the kidney.

115 (a) The ECG shows fast atrial fibrillation.
(b) There is no direct relationship between atrial fibrillation and high blood pressure, but patients with ischaemic heart disease or those who drink excessively are much more likely to develop atrial fibrillation. High blood pressure is a factor in the development of ischaemic heart disease and may be caused by excessive alcohol intake.

116 This M-mode echocardiogram shows severe concentric left ventricular hypertrophy in that there is a large increase in the thickness of the intraventricular septal wall and the posterior wall. This man had severe

hypertension which had remained untreated for many years prior to being seen.

117 (a) The ECG shows complete heart block and right bundle branch block.
(b) The complete heart block was precipitated by the use of a beta-blocker for this patient's high blood pressure. The beta-blocker was stopped but, in fact, in this patient the complete heart block persisted and he required permanent pacing.

118 (a) This is a maculopapular, measles-like rash.
(b) It is typical of the rashes that occurred with ACE inhibitors, particularly captopril, when given in high dosage. It is rare to see this rash now with the much lower doses of these drugs that are used.

119 These are typical, yellowish palmar striae lipid deposits. This is a rare finding and usually indicates severe hyperlipoproteinaemia and premature vascular disease.

120 There is a large intracerebral haemorrhage, and it can be seen that this was due to a large aneurysm that has burst.

121 These experiments, which have been carried out in three different strains of inherited hypertension in rats – the Dahl, the Milan, and the spontaneously hypertensive rat, have demonstrated that kidney transplant from a hypertensive strain rat to a normotensive strain rat results in hypertension in the transplanted rat. This is so even if the transplant is done before the hypertensive strain rat has developed hypertension. When the experiment is reversed – that is, the hypertensive strain rat has its kidneys removed and a normotensive kidney transplanted – the hypertensive rat no longer develops high blood pressure. These experiments clearly

demonstrate that, in these strains of inherited hypertension in the rat, the kidney carries the underlying message for the high blood pressure. Along with other circumstantial evidence, they demonstrate that the kidney may carry the primary fault for the development of high blood pressure in human essential hypertension.

122 (a) There is a marked corneal arcus.

(b) In older subjects there is controversy as to whether this in any way reflects vascular disease. It is certainly not related to high blood pressure, but in younger patients it may suggest abnormal blood lipids and a high fat intake, which will predispose to premature vascular disease.

123 (a) This patient had a phaeochromocytoma in the bladder.

(b) She presented with haematuria, and during cystoscopy was noticed by the anaesthetist to have extremely high blood pressure. Subsequent investigation revealed that she had a phaeochromocytoma in the bladder as shown in the MIBG scan and the CT scan of the pelvis. On further questioning she had noticed that when she strained to defecate or pass urine she experienced sweating, palpitations, and feelings of anxiety. The phaeochromocytoma was removed and it has not recurred during follow-up. Her blood pressure is now normal.

124 This is a typical rash caused by a dihydropyridine calcium antagonist, which occurs particularly in females.

125 (a) The retinal changes are those of severe hypertension. There are flame-shaped haemorrhages lying in the retina and filling the pattern of nerve fibre bundles going towards the disc. There are also cotton wool spots, which

are white and fluffy with indeterminate borders. The disc is normal. Retinal pigment epithelium is dark.

(b) The red colour is dull and, in view of his severe hypertension and retinal appearances, it could be assumed that this patient is Afro-Caribbean in origin.

(c) He was a 35-year-old male with accelerated hypertension without papilloedema. His blood pressure at presentation was 236/144 mm Hg.

126 There is severe narrowing in a coronary artery, which on cross-section can be seen to be due to a fibrous plaque that has ruptured with a thrombosis. This is the major cause of death in the Western world. High blood pressure is an important risk factor for the development of coronary artery disease.

Numbers refer to Question/Answer numbers